Male Yeast Infections

How to Diagnose, Treat and Cure Your Yeast Infection So it Never Comes Back

Bryan Cox

Male Yeast Infection Cures

Copyright © 2009 by Bryan Cox

Printed in the United States of America

For more information please visit:
www.MaleYeastInfectionCures.com

Contents

Introduction

Your body is filled with bacteria. Sounds a bit like a problem but really, there are good bacteria and bad bacteria and a bit of both are absolutely necessary to fight infection and create harmony in your body. A yeast infection is often seen as a female problem but in reality a lot of men don't realize that the yeast in their body might be having a very negative impact on their health.

Yeast infections are most often associated with being a female problem. In fact, almost as many men experience yeast problems as women. Yeast infections, also known as candida infections include several different types of infections and they affect men and women. This book, unlike most other yeast / candida guides, was written specifically for men so that men who deal with yeast problems can both understand the problem and find a solution that fits their life.

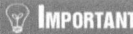 **IMPORTANT**

Is it a candida infection or a yeast infection? Yeast infections are also known as candida infections. There are many different species of candida yeasts. This book uses the terms candida infection and yeast infection interchangeably.

Yeast Infections: An Increasing Problem for Men

Candida is often ignored by men. Despite stereotypes, it just isn't true that men don't care about their health but because yeast is often thought of as a female issue, a lot of men that deal with these problems don't realize that they can learn to manage their body's bacteria levels so that the bacteria does its job instead of overpowering their life.

There's a saying that most women have at least one yeast infection in their lifetime. It would be more accurate to say that most people have a candida problem at some time in their lives. In some cases, people have the problem repeatedly. A lot of men can't figure out why they are continually plagued with recurring yeast infections but this book can help with: identifying yeast infections, identifying what to do about them and it might also be able to help you identify triggers in your own body for yeast overgrowth so that you can proactively work to stop this problem from recurring in the future.

Many males deal with various types of yeast infections and a lot of them deal with symptoms that are actually yeast-related without their even realizing it. You might be astonished when reading this book at some of the symptoms that can manifest as a result of yeast overgrowth.

There are many types of male yeast infections, many causes and treatment options. This book will share information about the various types of infections and various approaches to treatment including:
- prescription
- over the counter
- holistic
- prevention

While candida bacteria are present and necessary in all our bodies, letting them replicate out of control is what causes problems. Sometimes this happens because of health conditions, because of medication or even because of lifestyle. Regardless of the type of yeast infection you have, this book aims to help you take control of your health and deal with candida bacteria effectively.

Here are the topics we'll look at:
- Types of male yeast infections
- Risk factors

- Symptoms
- Diagnosis
- Prescription treatments
- Natural remedies
- Preventative measures
- Action plans

What will this book do for you?

This book will help you understand the causes and treatments for various yeast infections that men face and will help you take control of your health. Candida is receiving a lot of attention in the media and in medical laboratories. This bacteria is increasingly connected to many health problems and issues that don't just present as a problem but instead present as a lack of energy and vitality. This is preventable when a person understands the cues in their body that tell them something is unbalanced.

A yeast overgrowth can mean more than a penile discharge, rash in the groin or discharge in the mouth. It can impact many areas of your health. This book will look at various yeast infections and will also look at the larger problem of chronic candida.

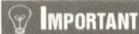 **IMPORTANT**

This book will also show you photographs of candida infections. Some of these photos are very graphic.

Yeast Infections that Affect Males

Why do we get yeast infections?

Yeast infections can happen for many reasons. Some of these reasons relate to other medical conditions. Sometimes it happens because of a weakened immune system. Certain medications we take can increase the chances of developing an infection and certain factors in our lifestyle can make us more susceptible.

Once you've had a yeast infection you can also be more prone to having recurring infections and over time might even recognize when a yeast infection is coming because of other factors in your life such as lifestyle and medication use. If you get yeast infections often you might get candida that is resistant to treatment. This can be a big problem but this book will help you address that.

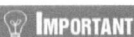 **IMPORTANT**

It's vital that you speak to your doctor if you have a yeast infection for the first time. Some other health conditions could mimic candida and until you know for a fact that this is not another health problem, it is not a good idea to simply self-treat as you could miss an important health diagnosis.

Is self treating candida ok?

In many cases, someone with recurring candida infections recognizes and is able to self-treat. Self-treatment can be effective but if you are dealing with recurring yeast infections it's important to determine the root cause and work to eliminate this problem.

Yeast: A Necessary Component

Men need yeast in their body. You do not want to eradicate candida altogether as it plays an important role in your health. Our bodies have many types of bacteria in them that work in many ways. But, when yeast colonizes to high levels, this is what creates an imbalance in the body. When they get to levels that exceed a healthy balance between positive and negative level of bacteria that's when health problems start.

Not all bacteria is bad bacteria.

Yeast lives in and on our bodies and plays an important role in our health. It is a fungus and can grow. When it grows in excess of the positive flora that helps regulate it, this is what causes problems. Those problems can be minor or they can even be life threatening.

For some men, a yeast infection is a nuisance. For others, it's hampering their life more than they realize. For many men, they don't even realise they have problems with their yeast levels which can be chronic. Some yeast infections can be deadly depending on your health and other medical issues. Because this is seen to be a female problem, many men don't even know they have it and because of that, they don't treat it or treat it with solutions that don't change the likelihood of recurring bouts. Candida can manifest itself in many ways and isn't always oral thrush or a rash.

Yeast is fungi and like bacteria, a fungus thrives in conditions that are favourable to them. Those who don't want yeast infection problems need to understand the favourable conditions that help yeast grow so they can change those conditions to unfavourable ones. Thankfully, what's unfavourable to yeast is favourable to good health so it is in your best interest to normalize the yeast levels in your body.

> **As far back as 1839 there are records of yeast problems being treated in terms of oral thrush.**

While yeast infections have been treated for generations, there is still much being learned about this fungus and continuing medical research reveals many ways to deal with it.

Types of Yeast

Various types of yeast exist and they can be divided in to four classes:

- Yeasts
- Yeast like fungi
- Moulds
- Dimorphic fungi

Although the term fungi encompass these four types, the term yeast is generally used to refer to candidal infection.

Candida infections and can refer to various types of yeast infections. There are 20 different species of candida but candida albicans is the most notable one.

To thrive, candida needs a host.

Candida bacterium doesn't thrive on its own. Candida depends on a living host for survival and is found living on us and in us. Candida species are normally found inhabiting the skin, mucosa (mouth, penis, vagina) and the intestines.

Candida colonizes in our mouths and throats and digestive system. Just because they are present does not mean they will cause problems but when they exceed typical numbers, then they become a problem and this happens most often when a person is in an ill state of health. This can happen for many reasons including a poor immune system or other medical conditions as well as the absence of health flora in the body that can regulate candida bacteria levels.

Secondary Candida Infections

Candida can cause secondary infection of other skin conditions like lichen planus and psoriasis. Candida infection is the most common fungal infection affecting persons with depressed immunity. Candida can be deadly to those with weak immune systems.

The Importance Of Positive Flora

Healthy flora in the body can help keep candida levels at a healthy balance. In addition to other areas explored, this book will talk about various ways to help you create and nurture positive flora in your body which can eliminate yeast infections and optimize digestive health.

If positive flora is destroyed, imagine it as law and order suddenly turning into rioting and looting or... a mutiny on a pirate ship.

Risk factors

Candida is commensal yeast which normally inhabits the body both inside and out. There are many beneficial microorganisms in these places and when the balance between these organisms and Candida gets disrupted, symptoms develop.

Not all males develop Candida infection. There are a few risk factors which predispose the person to the development of Candida infection.

The risk factors include:

- Intake of steroids – Steroids are drugs which suppress your body's immune system and this can cause yeast infections
- Use of antibiotics – Broad spectrum antibiotics like tetracycline don't just kill the body's harmful bacteria, they kill the beneficial bacteria (flora) as well. This imbalance causes candida levels to grow to levels that cause a yeast infection
- Severe trauma – Trauma breaches the protective skin or mucous membrane barrier allowing yeast to spread
- Catheterization of the bladder- This breaches the protective internal barrier that can allow existing yeast from the perineum (in the groin area) to enter the urinary tract and cause infection
- Blood cancers – These suppress immunity predisposing to yeast infection

- Bone marrow and solid organ transplantation – These suppress immunity predisposing to yeast infection
- Immunosuppressive disease like AIDS – This suppress immunity predisposing to yeast infection
- Wearing dentures – This causes damage to the mucosal lining allowing yeast to spread
- Smoking – Smoking increases the chances of yeast infection by 30-70%

Diet and lifestyle. Sedentary lifestyle and poor eating or hygiene habits can cause unhealthy bacteria to thrive and outnumber positive bacteria.

Candida transforms from a necessary factor in our bodies and becomes pathogenic when it invades the body due to excess numbers. Many factors can impact candida's ability to grow.

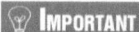 **IMPORTANT**

Creating a favourable environment for candida increases the problems and the likelihood of recurring infection.

Signs and Symptoms

Candida can affect the skin, mucous membrane and the internal organs. In males in addition to the penis, Candida can affect other parts of the body as well. Candida infection can cause ulcerative lesions affecting the mucous membrane in the mouth as well and this is called candidal or monilial stomatitis. There are various forms of monilial stomatitis which can affect males.

Oral thrush

Oral thrush is a fungal mouth infection due to Candida overgrowth. When Candida albicans gets colonized along the lining of the mouth it can result in white patches that resemble cottage cheese. These patches are extremely painful and make eating and drinking difficult. This condition, which is most common in babies, can affect adult males and most often affects elderly and chronically ill men. If you try to wipe the white patch off, it is painful and causes bleeding.

Oral thrush can develop suddenly and persist for a long time if left untreated. In severe cases, the oral thrush may spread to the back of the mouth and down through the throat.

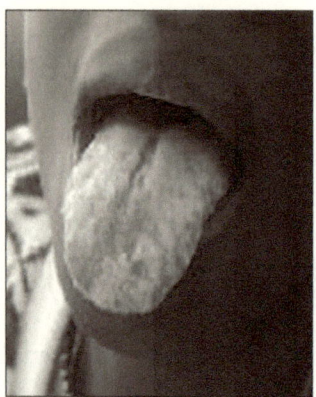

Figure 1: Image showing oral thrush

Acute hypertrophic candidiasis

In this condition, the tongue is most affected and a thick confluent lesion is found on the upper surface of the tongue. This often accompanies the onset of AIDS.

Acute atrophic candidiasis

This condition is most often seen as a complication of treatment with antibiotics. Again it is the tongue which is most affected. The sides of the upper surface of the tongue become smooth and red and the patient complains of a burning sensation.

Chronic atrophic candidiasis

This is also called denture sore mouth. In this condition a red swollen mucosa is produced over the area covered by an upper denture. Despite being called "denture sore mouth", this condition is usually painless. The patient's denture hygiene is generally poor and needs to be improved. Further, the patients often wear dentures at night which exacerbates the problem.

Chronic hypertrophic candidiasis

In this condition the mucosal lining becomes thick which is hard and rough to the touch. Lesions usually occur on the inner sides of the cheeks and sometimes on the tongue. The lesions appear as speckled white on a pink background rather than uniform white. This is also called speckled leukoplakia and it often affects smokers. Those who develop speckled leukoplakia are particularly prone to developing cancer.

Chronic mucocutaneous candidiasis

This candida infection is a disorder of the immune system. These patients develop extensive yeast infection of the skin, mucous membrane and the nails.

Angular cheilitis

This is also called perleche and angular stomatitis. These are reddish fissures in the angle of the mouth. Candida infection is one of the causes of angular cheilitis and this is common in those who take the drug Isotretinoin for the treatment of acne.

Median rhomboid glossitis

This is a diamond shaped inflammation of the back of the tongue which results due to a yeast infection.

Exfoliative cheilitis

In this condition, the yeast infection causes peeling of the surface of the lips. This is usually seen in patients with the HIV infection.

Balanitis (Yeast infection of penis)

Balanitis is the infection of the penis and can happen as a result of a male having sex with someone with a vaginal yeast infection. This type of candida also occurs due to irritants and overgrowth of organisms that are normally present on the skin of the penis which includes Candida.

Balanitis is most common in patients who are affected by diabetes mellitus. In many cases, patients consult their doctor for the symptoms of balanitis and during the course of the investigation, diabetes is sometimes diagnosed. This further demonstrates why it's important that candida infections do not simply get self-treated or ignored.

Self treating or ignoring chronic Candida could mean you're overlooking another health problem such as HIV/AIDS or Diabetes

Other risk factors are:

- Uncircumcised men with poor personal hygiene are the most affected by balanitis. Balanitis is a common condition affecting 11% of adult men seen in urology clinics in the US. Balanitis may occur in up to 3% of uncircumcised males worldwide.
- Poor personal hygiene
- Chemical irritants like soap
- Obesity

If the foreskin is moist and not cleaned for a couple of days, the above risk factors predispose the person to yeast infection of the penis resulting in balanitis. In most of the patients the only symptoms is itching of the penis.

The other symptoms include:
- Discharge from the affected part
- Redness
- Swelling of the affected part
- Painful foreskin with exuding pus
- Inability to retract the foreskin in severe cases

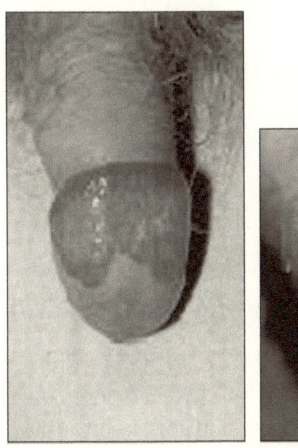 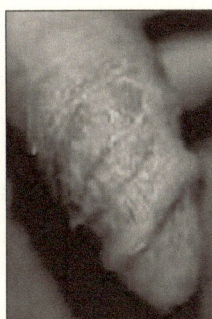

Figure 2: Images showing balanitis

The diagnosis is usually confirmed by culturing the pus and taking a smear of the lesion and examining it under the microscope for the presence of yeast organisms. If balanitis is not treated properly it may result in phimosis. Phimosis is a condition in which the foreskin of the penis cannot be retracted.

Candidal intertrigo

Intertrigo is a condition in which skin surface or the skin folds get inflamed due to infection. Candidal infection is one of the common causes of intertrigo. Candidal intertrigo can affect different parts of the body. Some of the commonly affected areas in males are:

Between the toes – This is called athlete's foot. This condition can also be caused by tinea, dermatitis and psoriasis. The skin is moist, white and peeling.

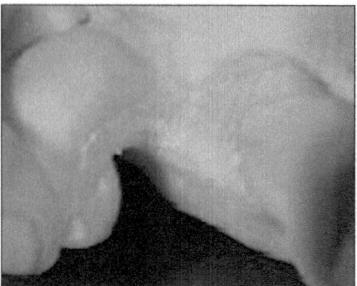

Figure 3: Image showing Candida infection between the toes

Web spaces of hand – Intertrigo of the web spaces of the hand occurs in persons whose occupation includes gardening. The hands of these individuals are wet and moist. The infection usually occurs during warm climates. The lesions appear moist, white, peeling and is very uncomfortable

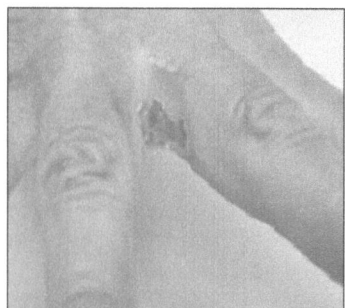

Figure 4: Image showing Candida infection of the web space of the hand

Groin, between the buttocks – These occur as a result of excess moisture. The affected areas show bright red lesions which are moist, cracked and sore. There are usually tiny surface "satellite" spots, blisters or pustules along the border of the lesions. The predisposing factors include obesity, hot weather, poor hygiene, tight clothing and use of topical steroids. Patients suffering from this condition usually complain of itching and burning.

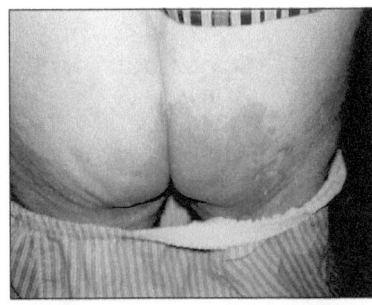
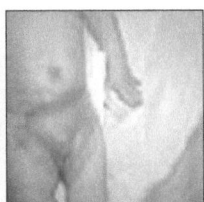

Figure 5: Image showing Candida infection of the groin and buttocks

The diagnosis is usually done by taking a scraping of the lesion and examining under microscope and also by culturing the material taken from the lesion.

Yeast infection of the nails

Candida can infect the nails. The condition affecting the nail fold is called paronychia and Candida causes chronic paronychia. Most often a mixture of yeasts and bacteria cause chronic paronychia. It is very difficult to cure chronic paronychia completely. Sometimes it occurs as a complication of eczema. Chronic mucocutaneous candidiasis affects the nail plate and eventually infects the proximal and lateral nail folds.

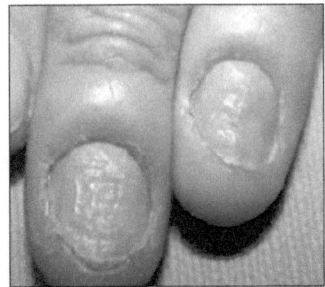

Figure 6: Image showing Candida infection of the nails

Chronic paronychia usually occurs during winter months. Chronic paronychia most often occurs in persons whose hands are repeatedly exposed to moist environments or in those who have prolonged and repeated contact with irritants such as mild acids, mild alkalis, or other chemicals. It mainly occurs in people who have constantly wet hands, such as dairy farmers, fishermen, bar tenders and housewives.

It usually starts in one nail. But it can spread to others. The affected nail fold is swollen and lifted of the nail plate. It is red and painful and pus may be expressed from under the fold. The nail plate becomes distorted and horizontal ridges are formed. The cuticles and nail folds may separate from the nail plate, forming a space for the invasion of various microorganisms. The symptoms usually last 6 weeks or longer. After treatment, it may take months for the nail to appear normal again.

Infection of the nail bed, nail plate or nail matrix is called onychomycosis. Toenails are much more likely to be infected than fingernails. 30% of patients with a cutaneous fungal infection also have onychomycosis.

The risk factors for development of onychomycosis include the following:

- Old age
- Diabetes
- Suppression of the immune system by diseases and drugs

Yeast infection of the nails can also cause onycholysis. Onycholysis is a condition in which nail is lifted from its bed. It may appear yellow or white and is usually painless as the separation occurs gradually. Pain may occur if nail is further detached from the nail bed as result of trauma or if active infection sets in.

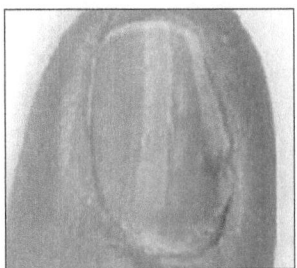

Figure 7: Image showing onycholysis

Yeast infection of food pipe

Yeast infection of the food pipe is also called as esophageal moniliasis. Candidal organisms are the most common food pipe infection even in people with strong immune systems.

It is estimated that up to 20% of normal healthy adults have colonization of the food pipe with Candida.

The risk factors of development of food pipe yeast infection are:

- Achalasia cardia – In this condition, the lower end of the food pipe does not open up to allow the food to enter the stomach. The food particles stay in the food pipe and this may result in yeast infection
- Scleroderma – In this condition, the wall of the food pipe is affected and the food pipe does not contract adequately to push the food bolus down. This result in retention of food particles in the food pipe and this may result in yeast infection.
- Topical steroids – Patients who take steroids using inhal-

ers especially for asthma may suffer from yeast infection of the oral cavity and the food pipe. The steroid particles get deposited on the surface resulting in yeast infection. This can be prevented by gargling after using the inhalers.

- Diabetes – This condition causes a suppression of the immune system resulting in yeast infection
- Old age- This again predisposes to yeast infection secondary to poor immunity

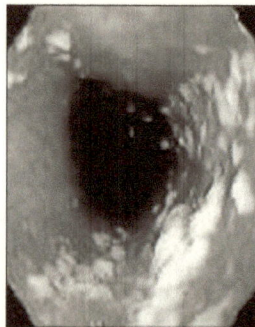
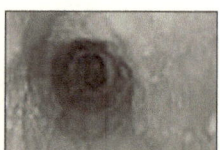

Figure 8: Images showing yeast infection of the food pipe

Symptoms of Food Pipe Candida

Food pipe yeast infection produces three symptoms.

1. The patient may have a sense of obstruction on swallowing,
2. They may have pain behind the breast bone while swallowing,
3. And, bleeding may occur.

In most of the cases this chest pain is wrongly attributed to heart disease. The lesions of food pipe yeast infection appear as areas of redness with swelling, discrete white patches or ulcers. Most of the lesions are seen in the lower third of the food pipe.

The diagnosis is usually done using the following methods:

- Endoscopy – Endoscopy allows direct visualization of the inner side of the food pipe and the Candida lesions. The lesions can be seen as per the description given above.
- Brushing –During endoscopy, brushing of the lesions is done and the material obtained is examined under microscope to visualize the Candida organisms
- Culture – In this procedure, the material obtained from the lesions is cultured in a special medium and growth of the organism is looked for.

In addition to the above conditions yeast can also cause infection deep inside the body. Some of the common deep yeast infections are:

Gastrointestinal yeast infection

Apart from food pipe yeast can also affect stomach, small intestine and the large intestine. The symptoms include abdominal pain, vomiting, bloating and abdominal mass and GI yeast infections often take over the whole body. This subject is discussed at length in this book.

Yeast infection of the vocal chord

This occurs especially in those with cancers

Yeast infection of the lungs

Lung candida is difficult to diagnose. The patient suffers from breathlessness, cough and fever.

Yeast infection of bladder

This can occur when the bladder is catheterized. The patient has burning during urination, blood in urine and feels urgency to urinate.

Yeast infection of the kidney

The use of stents and indwelling devices, along with the presence of diabetes, is the major risk factor predisposing patients to yeast infection of the kidneys. The patient complains of pain, vomiting, fever and blood in urine.

Yeast infection of the liver and spleen

This usually occurs in having cancer or AIDS. The symptoms include: fever, not responding to antibiotics, abdominal pain, abdominal distension and on occasion: jaundice

Yeast infection of the heart

The risk factors include intravenous heroin use, which is frequently associated with infection due to *Candida parapsilosis,* chemotherapy; prosthetic valves (approximately 50%) and prolonged use of central venous catheters.

Yeast infection of the eyes

Factors responsible for yeast infection of eye are eye injury, eye surgery. The patients complain of pain in the eyes, fever, floating objects in the field of vision.

Yeast infection of the brain

This is very difficult to diagnose and treat. The symptoms include fever, neck rigidity, confusion and coma

Yeast infection of the joints

This may be caused by injury and through blood spread.

As you can see, candida is a condition that can impact many areas of the body and your health.

Chronic Candidiasis

Chronic candidasis can happen when yeast is running rampant in your body and in this case you might not even know you have candida. Some people don't have rashes or a discharge but have many other symptoms that are akin to feeling run down and sluggish. Candida feasts on sugar so most often thrives in an unhealthy body. If your pH level is low, for instance, Candida can spread and a pH test can be a good indicator of whether or not your bacteria levels are out of sync.

Those with candida overgrowth often have a poor diet and sedentary lifestyle. Here are some of the symptoms associated with chronic or systemic candida infections:

- Digestive problems
- Lethargy and fatigue
- Mood swings / depression
- Low sex drive

- Food cravings
- Feeling bloated
- Lack of ability to concentrate
- Weight gain
- Developing food allergies
- Acne
- Hives
- Other symptoms listed in this book

You might have a rash, you might not. You might have some of these symptoms or you might have them all. Our bodies are strong and robust but when they go off balance it can create a domino affect that might impact one person in one way and someone else in an entirely different manner.

Diagnosis

Although Candida can cause a number of different forms of diseases of the skin, mucous membrane and the internal organs, there are a few basic investigations which may help in the diagnosis of a yeast infection. The basis of all investigations is to demonstrate the presence of yeast. The various investigations include:

- Direct microscopy
- Culture
- Blood tests
- Home tests

Collection of Specimen

This is done by the following methods.

- Scraping from the edge of the lesion
- Hair along with its root
- Brushings from the lesion
- Nail clippings
- Skin biopsy
- Moist swab from the mucosal surface

Direct Microscopy

In this method, the collected specimen is examined directly under the microscope for the presence of yeast organisms. As Candida can be seen on normal skin or mucosa as well, only their abundant presence is of significance. The success rate of finding candida overgrowth through this method includes:

- 10% Potassium hydroxide preparation(KOH) stained with blue or black ink
- Unstained wet mount
- Using special stains like Periodic Acid Schiff (PAS) and methanamine silver stains

Under microscope yeast organisms can be identified with the following features –

- Round or ovoid cells
- Presence of branched filaments. Presence of mycelium indicates colony formation and tissue invasion

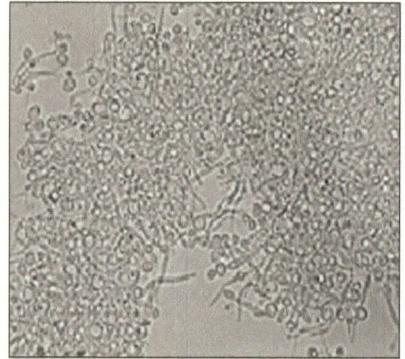

Figure 9: Microscopic image of Candida

Culture

The specimen collected is cultured in a special medium and growth of yeast organisms are looked for. The culture process is done at 25 – 30⁰ C and it may take several weeks for the yeast to grow. The culture media that are commonly used include Sabouraud's glucose agar, Czapek-Dox medium and Cornmeal agar. Cycloheximide is added to the medium to prevent contamination with moulds. Colonies of yeast organisms appear creamy white, smooth and with smell like yeast.

Blood tests

Unlike in bacteria infections blood tests are seldom helpful in diagnosing the yeast infection. Yeast infection may be diagnosed by demonstrating the presence of antigens and antibodies in blood.

There are a few additional tests which are done along with the above mentioned tests in the diagnosis of yeast infections. They are:
- Urine analysis in yeast infection of kidney and urinary bladder
- The serum 1-3 D-glucan detection assay to measure the level of fungal wall component
- Gastrointestinal endoscopy to visualize the lesion and to collect the specimen for examination
- Bronchoscopy to visualize the lesion in the respiratory tract and to collect the specimen for examination
- Serum alkaline phosphatase levels to diagnose yeast infection of liver
- Chest x-ray to diagnose pneumonia caused by yeast
- Ultra sonogram and CT scan for diagnosing yeast infection of liver, spleen and kidney
- Echocardiography for diagnosing yeast infection of the lining of the heart

Home-Based Tests

Saliva Test

If you want to test yourself for Candida, you can spit into a glass of water as soon as you wake up in the morning. Check every few minutes for the appearance of the saliva for up to an hour. If the water is fairly clear you probably don't have a candida overgrowth but if cloudy substances, stringy substances or specks appear in the glass there's a good chance you have excess yeast in your body.

PH Test

A pH balance test can be done at home and those with very acidic levels (below 7) often have candida infections. You can buy paper kits that you can test with saliva or urine to determine your pH level.

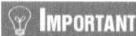 **IMPORTANT**

Home tests can reveal candida presence but many doctors suggest you still speak with a doctor before self-treating your first case of candida.

Effective Treatment

Yeast infections are often less harmful when compared to bacterial infections. But treating a yeast infection can be very difficult. It's important to treat all yeast infections whether you choose to treat them with medicine from the pharmacy, a prescription from your doctor or holistic / natural treatment. It may take long period of time for complete cure and recurrence of the disease is common but the knowledge throughout this book can help you reduce or eliminate the recurrence of yeast infections.

The treatment of yeast infections can be divided in to the following categories.

- General measures
- Medical management
- Surgical management
- Natural cures

General measures

The general measures including self care at home and this helps in faster cure of the yeast infection and also it helps in preventing any further yeast infection. The various measures that are to be taken are:

- The risk factors which predispose the person to yeast infection should be treated. For example diabetes is a very common risk factor which may cause yeast infection in the affected patient. If diabetes is treated and blood glucose is controlled, yeast infection can be easily treated and prevented.

- Moistness is one of the important causes of yeast infection. So the skin has to be kept dry to prevent yeast infection. Yeast infection is common between skin folds. So skin fold have to be kept dry.

- Clothes should be washed at a temperature of at least 60^0 C

- Towels should not be shared with others.

- Open toed slippers should be worn

- Tight dressing should be avoided

- Dentures should be cleaned regularly and good oral hygiene maintained

- If the patient is affected with yeast infection of the genitals, its better to avoid sex until it is treated. Or he can use a condom to protect the spread of the infection to his partner. Also if the female partner is infected, he can use a condom to protect himself from getting infected. But if yeast creams are used it is better to avoid the latex condoms as they can break. The best thing to get faster relief and to prevent spread to partners is abstaining from sexual activity. In case of infection both the partners need to be treated for optimum results.

- Unnecessary use of antibiotics especially the broad spectrum antibiotics like tetracycline should be avoided whenever possible. When antibiotics need to be taken, the patient should take good care to follow a sensible diet and consider probiotic foods which create healthy flora and prebiotic food to nurture flora.

- A well balanced diet will boost the immunity and prevent yeast infection
- Many foods should be avoided. More on this will be explored in this book
- Deodorants and body sprays should be avoided as these can irritate the skin

Medical treatment

Medical treatment consists of medications which can cure yeast infection. These drugs are available as both topical which has to be applied on the lesion and oral medication which has to be taken by mouth.

Topical drugs

There are various topical drugs available to treat yeast infections.

For skin infections:

The topical drugs are to be applied on the affected areas twice a day. While applying the cream several centimeters of normal skin around the lesion also should be included. The treatment has to be continued for typically 2-4 weeks but always follow the directions otherwise the bacteria can grow again and become resistant to that treatment method in future. The treatment should typically be continued for at least 2 weeks after the last visible rash disappears.

- Whitfield ointment
- Ciclopirox olamine
- Nystatin
- Clotrimazole

- Miconozole
- Ketaconazole
- Econozole
- Tioconazole
- Undecylenic alkanolamide
- Terbenafine
- Tolciclate
- Tolfnatatearound the lseion o be applied on the lesion and oral mfected patient. yeast infection.

For nail fold infections:

Treatment often occurs twice daily for a couple of months.
- 3% Thymol in chloroform
- 5% Sulfacetamide in spirit
- Econozole
- Miconozole

For nail plate infection:

Mild nail plate infections can be treated with topical medication applied once or twice weekly. The affected nail should be roughened initially with an emery board and the medication is then applied on it. The preparations available are -
- Morpholine
- Ciclopirox olamine

Best results can be expected:
- If less than 80% of the nail plate is infected
- If the growing part of the nail plate is not involved
- If there is no existing internal disease like diabetes or skin disease like psoriasis

For mouth infections

The following preparations are typically used to treat oral thrush:
- Miconozole
- Nystatin
- Amphotericin B

Oral drugs

Oral drugs are used if the yeast infection is severe or if there is not a good response to topical treatment. The choice of the drugs depends on several factors including the site of infection, presence of other diseases and interaction with other drugs.

Options include:
- Itraconazole
- Ketaconazole
- Fluconazole
- Voriconazole
- Nystatin
- Flucytosine
- Amphotericin B

The treatment of yeast infections under special circumstances are as follows:
- In HIV positive patients, the response may be poor. In these cases in addition to treating HIV infection, yeast infection is treated with higher dosage of fluconazole or itraconazole.
- Food pipe yeast infection needs treatment for 14-21 days with fluconazole or itraconazole
- In yeast infection of urinary bladder in patients who

have a urinary catheter, changing the catheter alone may sometimes cure the infection. In patients without catheter drugs (fluconazole) are to be given for 14-21 days.

- In case of the yeast organisms developing resistance to the drugs, higher dose of the drugs are to be given or can be treated with the following –
    - Caspofungin
    - Lipid preparations of amphotericin B
    - Voriconazole
    - A combination of amphotericn B and flucystosine
    - Human recombinant monoclonal antibody

Surgical treatment

Surgical treatment is not a typical treatment for yeast infection and generally only happens when there is:

- Yeast infection of the spleen
- Yeast infection of the breast bone or the spine
- Yeast infection of the inner lining of the heart may require valve replacement surgery
- Yeast infection of joint prosthesis may require removal of the prosthesis

Home Remedies and Natural Cures

Home remedies and natural cures can be tried in milder yeast infections. But if the patient is doubtful about the diagnosis or if the infection is severe you need to see a doctor before attempting to cure it on your own.

Some people prefer holistic remedies over the "over the counter" or "prescribed" options because they feel safer about using natural products. Many natural products work at not only treating symptoms and curing the problem but many can be taken proactively as part of health and wellness to keep candida levels under control.

And, home remedies such as the below are often used after a patient has developed a resistance to specific drugs because of overuse. This is a good case for learning about your candida because if you are getting it so often that drugs are becoming ineffective it's time to look further than the symptoms. It's time to look at the root of your candida problems.

Again, you should always be aware of what you are dealing with. Self-treating can carry the risk of missing a problem. When a natural remedy works, it's usually indicative of resolution but if the symptoms continually worsen, it's wise to see your doctor.

Some of the commonly used home remedies are as follows. Not all of these will work for everyone but you may find options here that can help you treat candida or prevent it from recurring.

Yogurt

Yogurt is one of the easily available home made remedies for the treatment of male yeast infections. On the surface of the body and in the intestine there are always a group of microorganisms who are beneficial for humans. These micro flora are destroyed by intake of broad spectrum antibiotics, injury and by diseases like AIDS and diabetes. This imbalance facilitates the growth of yeast.

Based on this, if you replace the beneficial microorganisms in your body, they can help you eliminate yeast overgrowth. Yogurt is one of the richest sources of these microorganisms due to the presence of lactophilus acidophilus, lactobacillus casei, bifidobacterium, streptococcus salivaricus and thermophilus.

These beneficial bacteria are called probiotics. You can buy probiotic yogurt in your grocery store and take it proactively when you're taking antibiotics or make it part of your regular diet. Many juices with probiotics are also available.

Yogurt can both cure and also prevent yeast infections. It can even help women with vaginal infections and many not only consume it but douche with it as well.

Acidophilus acts on lactose and other nutrients and breaks them down in to lactic acid, hydrogen peroxide and other related products. These products are acidic in nature and they change the body to a state of being inhospitable for yeast growth. Acidophilus is involved in the production of vitamins like niacin, folic acid and pyridoxine which are involved in many chemical reactions resulting in cell repair, energy production and boosting of immunity. Acidophilus also consumes nutrients on which the harmful bacteria are dependent and make them deprived of those nutrients.

There are a few studies which confirm these beneficial effects of lactobacillus in the treatment of Candida infection. Zwolinska et al from the department of Gastroenterology, Poland conducted a study on this and have concluded that these probiotics are effective in the treatment of fungal colonization of the gastrointestinal tract and they shorten the duration of the colonization of Candida in the gut (Source: Journal of Physiology and Pharmacology, 2006 Nov;57 Supplement 9:35-49). Similar observations are made by Mazzoni from Department of Neonatology, Italy (Source: Clinical Infectious Diseases, 2006 Jun 15; 42(12):1735-42) and Wagner from The Department of Medical Microbiology (Source: Journal of Food Protection. 2000 May; 63(5):638-44).

Garlic

Garlic is known for many medicinal properties including a cure for candida. It is also called as 'Allium sativum'. Garlic contains many helpful compounds like allicin, diallyl disulphide, vitamin C, vitamin B6, selenium and manganese.

Garlic has strong antibiotic properties and complete absence of development of resistance to microorganisms so unlike some bacterial medications your candida won't grow immune to garlic. Garlic juice is bactericidal at concentrations of 5% and more. Fresh garlic extract has a greater efficacy than garlic powder extracts so using fresh garlic whenever possible as well as taking garlic pills (which can help eliminate the odor) can be very helpful. If cooking garlic, avoid boiling it for more than 5 minutes during cooking for optimal results.

Date extracts

Dates are edible fruits of Palm dates that are mainly grown in desert regions. Dates are well known for medicinal properties and are used as infusions, decoction, syrup and paste. The medicinal properties of dates are attributed to high tannin and iron content. Many studies have shown that date extracts are very effective in the prevention of yeast infections.

Date extracts are very helpful with oral thrush because they prevent this adherence of yeast to the lining of the mouth. (Source: Journal of Oral Pathology and Medicine, 2000 May; 29(5):200-5) and can cause weakening or collapse of the fungi's cell wall.

Honey

Honey is a powerful home remedy for many health issues. It has many components such as vitamin B6, vitamin C, thiamin, niacin, riboflavin, pantothenic acid, calcium, copper, iron, magnesium, manganese, phosphorus, potassium, sodium, and zinc as well as several different amino acids. Honey has been used for its medicinal properties for more than 2500 years. The anti-microbial effects of honey are due to low water activity, hydrogen peroxide activity and high acidity. Honey increases the amount of beneficial bacteria (probiotics) in the intestine and can strengthen your immune system.

Tea tree oil

Tea-tree oil is often referred to as first aid in a bottle and it has received much attention as a natural remedy for bacterial and fungal infections of the skin and mucosa. Several published studies have recently demonstrated tea-tree oil's antibacterial and anti-fungal activities.

Tea tree oil is also called Melaleuca oil and should only be used only for external application for yeast. About 10% of people show allergy to this oil but most people tolerate it well.

Tree tea oil is found to be effective even in drug resistant yeast infections (Source: BMC Infectious Diseases, 2006 Nov 3; 6:158). In fact, it is recently being looked at as an alternative regimen for advanced HIV-positive patients with oropharyngeal candidiasis refractory to fluconazole.

Pau d'arco bark

Pau d'arco is obtained from the bark of a South American tree. It has been broadly used as ornamental tree in landscaping gardens, public squares and boulevards due to its impressive and colorful flowering. The inner bark is dried, shredded and then boiled making a bitter or sour-tasting brownish-colored tea. It is also available in pill form. Its main active principles are lapachol, quercetin and other flavonoids.

Pau d'arco bark has anti-yeast properties and when boiled for ten to twenty minutes is given in teaspoon form two or three times a day and often used with vinegar in a bath as well.

Boric acid

Boric acid is a mild acid used as an anti-septic agent. Boric acid can be used to treat yeast and fungal infections and is especially useful in the treatment of resistant yeast infections. Boric acid is effective in curing 98% of the patients who had previously failed to respond to the most commonly used antifungal agents and is clearly indicated as the drug of choice for prevention of yeast infections. Some yeast require more Boric Acid than others. For instance, Candida glabrata requires higher concentrations than Candida albicans.

Boric acid seems to be a valid and promising therapy both in the cure of the and in the prevention of relapses of recurrent yeast infections but once stopping usage relapses are common.

Gentian violet

Gentian violet is a dye which is used as an anti-yeast agent. It is also called as crystal violet, methyl violet 10B and hexamethyl pararosaniline chloride. It is painted on skin or gums to treat or prevent fungal infections. Gentian violet does not require a doctor's prescription but can stain the cloth and has been linked to cancer in the digestive tract of some animals. It is usually used as weak solutions either as 1% or 2% solutions.

Kefir

Kefir is a fermented milk drink. It is prepared with cow, goat, or sheep's milk with kefir grains. Kefir grains are a combination of bacteria and yeasts in a matrix of proteins, lipids, and sugars. The result is a sour, carbonated, slightly alcoholic beverage, with a consistency similar to thin yogurt. Kefir can be considered a probiotic source as it presents anti-bacterial, anti-mycotic, and anti-neoplastic and immunomodulatory properties. A total of 21 strains of Lactobacillus species have been isolated from Turkish kefir samples and lactophilus as mentioned earlier are very effective in curing yeast infections. Taking this product can significantly increase the beneficial bacteria in your body.

Berberine extracts

Berberine is a plant alkaloid found in herbs such as berberis, goldenseal, and coptis chinensis. It is effective against fungal infections, candida, yeast, parasites, bacterial and viral infections. Both methanolic extract and alkaloidal fraction of Berberis aetnensis are effective against Candida species. Synthetic products of berberine also are available. The synthesized compounds exhibit more potent antifungal activities than berberine and berberrubine. Berberine is particularly useful in the treatment drug resistant yeast infections and it also helps to facilitate effectiveness of the drug amphotericin B.

Olive leaf extract

Olive is a small tree of the Mediterranean region. Olive leaves are used in medicinal teas. According to research, they have anti-yeast properties and 15% (w/v) olive plant extract can kill yeast within 24 hours. Scanning electron microscopic observations of candida albicans that were exposed to 40% (w/v) olive leaf extract, showsdistorted cells. These findings suggest an anti-yeast potential of olive leaves.

Coconut Oil

Caprylic acid is a fatty acid. It is present in coconut and breast milk.

It is an oily liquid with a slightly unpleasant rancid taste that is minimally soluble in water. Caprylic acid is known to have anti-fungal properties, and is often recommended by nutritionists for the treatment of yeast infections.

It is especially useful for treating infection of the gut. When using coconut oil you can consume it on its own and you can also cook with it. It cooks beautifully as it has a high melting point so food doesn't burn the way it does when frying with other oils. Food doesn't have to taste like coconut, either as coconut oil doesn't typically have a coconut flavor.

Oil of Oregano

Oregano is high in antioxidant activity, due to a high content of phenolic acids and flavonoids. It's also an antibacterial / antiseptic and fungus and germs do not become immune to it so this is an ideal solution for improving your immune system. This is not typical oregano found in your spice rack but extracted oil from oregano.

Apple Cider Vinegar

Apple cider vinegar is a popular folk remedy for many conditions including yeast. Organic apple cider vinegar that's not pasteurized contains a cloudy substance known as the 'mother'. While regular vinegar isn't recommended in the diet of those trying to starve their candida bacteria, this type of vinegar can actually help treat and prevent yeast infections. It can help with pH level, with digestive functions and the body's immune system which creates an inhospitable environment for candida albicans bacteria.

Breathing and Meditation

Breathing is cleansing for the body and the soul. Stress can cause havoc in your body whereas relaxation is actually cleansing. Those who practice deep breathing and meditation reduce stress in their bodies and their minds and this is very healthy for the body. Correct breathing can even lower blood pressure in people who have dangerously high blood pressure. Oxygenating your body and your blood improves your immune system and candida thrives in an area with lack of oxygen.

Colon Health

Yeast thrives in toxic conditions and when your colon isn't operating at full capacity, this gives yeast an ideal breeding ground. When our digestive systems are sluggish, bacteria and fungus will grow exponentially.

Slow colon transit time creates toxicity in the body so colon cleansing and regularity will help your body's pH balance and your immune system as well as keep the healthy bacteria thriving and the unhealthy yeast at a minimum. Eat plenty of fiber and increase your colon transit time through healthful eating.

Laxatives aren't suggested for optimum colon health because you can become dependent on them but natural fiber through healthy eating will increase colon transit time and reduce candida and other bacteria build up in your digestive tract.

Exercise

Exercise oxygenates the body but yeast thrives in a sluggish environment or body. The more oxygenated your body, the better for you and the worse for yeast. That's why breathing exercises can help as well as aerobic exercises. Sweating also removes toxins from your body which improves your immune system and your body's balance.

Even mild exercise such as walking or swimming or low-impact such as jumping on a rebounder can be very effective in helping you to reduce yeast in your body. Exercise creates energy and the more energetic you are, the less hospitable you are to candida. Of course you'll need to be sure you dry yourself well after exercising and swimming, especially if you're prone to yeast rashes.

Water

Water is obviously essential to everyone but if you increase your water intake you can make a difference to your body's methods of processing food and toxins. This is especially helpful when you've eaten something unhealthy. Drinking plenty of water also increases your colon transit time.

A Preventative Diet

A good way to eradicate candida from your body is to starve it out. Unhealthy yeast crave yeast foods and they like sugar. Removing sugar and yeast from your diet is a wise way to starve candida so they cannot thrive.

Foods To Avoid

Avoid foods like: mushrooms, any refined sugars, enriched white bread and cereal, pasta, vinegar and beer. *(Beer? Sugar? I know what you're thinking! But keep reading. You don't necessarily have to give up beer and sweets forever.)*

Foods To Consume

Feed your body with probiotics, prebiotics, whole grains, vegetables and lean protein.

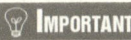 **IMPORTANT**

Ezekiel 4:9 bread is a flourless, sprouted grain bread that's known to be helpful to yeast sufferers. The name comes from a Bible passage that describes the recipe.

Probiotics and Prebiotics

As mentioned, probiotics provide healthy flora for your body and can aid with digestion. You can also take prebiotics which act as food for your healthy flora. Beyond buying cheese and juice that has prebiotics in it, a good example of prebiotics would be: foods with inulin such as chicory, artichokes, onions, garlic. A symbiotic such as kefir contains both pre and pro biotics.

A synbiotic is a supplement that contains both pre and probiotics.

Those looking to fight candida often find that doing a candida diet for several weeks can make a big difference. They can then gradually reintroduce the foods they've been avoiding in low quantities and with the presence of other healthy foods. For instance, if you are concerned that you can no longer drink beer, this isn't necessarily the case.

Candida and Beer or Wine

Once you have your candida issues resolved you can drink beer or wine without concern provided that most of your health and life style habits are good ones. Because so many factors impact yeast levels, if most of your habits are good ones and you are in overall good health you'll be able to indulge in sugar in your coffee or a few beers on the weekends.

Your Action Plan

Your candida action plan can be reactive and proactive so that not only will you regulate the yeast levels in your body but that you'll also prevent recurrences of overgrowth.

This book's aim is to help you understand why candida might be in your life, help you look at various treatment options and help you prevent it from recurring and you can use the information you've read here to take control of your health.

Here's an action plan for ridding candida from your life.
1. Identify the presence of excess yeast.
2. Treat
3. Prevent

Once you identify this is a problem you need to treat it. You can treat it at the doctor's office through medication and you can sometimes treat it holistically at home. The prevention part is key and lifestyle changes can help you prevent it from recurring.
- Diet changes
- Probiotic supplements
- Exercise
- Drinking enough water
- Bowel movement regularity

- Reducing stress
- Getting in tune with your body

Getting in tune with your body becomes easier as you explore your health and learn how to strengthen your immune system. You might find that a daily dose of apple cider vinegar, using coconut oil in your food and eating yogurt a few times a week helps keep candida away permanently. This might not be enough for you.

You might decide to eliminate sugar from your diet altogether and maybe to take an oil of oregano supplement. Or, you might find that another mixture of treatments works for you. It's important that you pay attention to your body's signals. It won't always be a penile yeast infection that alerts you that something is off. You might just start feeling sluggish or moody all of a sudden.

Or, you might find patches of white in your mouth. Whatever your individual situation, the advice in this book can help you overcome not just candida but can help you improve your lifestyle so that you take control of your health and improve your energy, your appearance and your longevity.

Bonus Articles

In an attempt to provide you with the most useful information possible we have included a bonus section.

This section contains additional material and articles to help you understand yeast infections even further and to help guide you in your quest to not only treat but cure your yeast infection problem.

Thank you for investing in this book and enjoy these bonus articles.

As a Male; How Could I Get a Yeast Infection?

Could I get, as a male, yeast infections of the sort that women often contract? I always thought those yeast infection were not male problems. But now I have a penile discharge and it is a little uncomfortable when I urinate. Is it possible that I have contracted a male yeast infection or is this something much worse?

If this sounds like something you have been thinking, you should know that even males of every age, race, and economic status, or physical prowess, can and often do experience male yeast infections. Now, you are probably wondering how you could get such a yeast infection.

There are two main ways that men get yeast infections. By far the most common means of contracting a penile yeast infection is having unprotected sex with a female that has an active vaginal yeast infection. The yeast bacteria in the vagina enter the penis and, in some cases, manage to multiple sufficiently to become a full-blow infection. The bacteria that cause a yeast infection are normally present in the human body, but the number of bacteria are maintain at a proper level by the good bacteria that live in our bodies.

Keep in mind, also, that unprotected sexual activity with another man can just as easily allow the transmission of a yeast infection. So, no matter what your sexual preference, practice safe sex!

The second most common cause of male yeast infection is prolonged use of antibiotic therapy for another medication problem.

When antibiotics are taken orally or by injection, the antibiotics kill bacteria. However, these medications are not smart; they can not tell which bacteria are beneficial to the body and which are causing illness or disease. The good bacteria which keep bad bacteria at bay are reduced to a level that yeast bacteria establish a stronghold and a male yeast infection occurs.

There are a few other rare ways in which a male can get a yeast infection. Unprotected anal sex, for example, puts a man at risk of a penile yeast problem. Wearing tight, damp clothing can, in rare cases, cause a man to experience a yeast outbreak.

Fortunately, if you have symptoms that indicate you might have a yeast infection in your penis or genital area, treatment is easy and effective. In many cases over the counter creams and ointments will clear up the yeast infection. These creams and ointments are the same ones recommended for women to combat vaginal yeast infections.

> ### 💡 IMPORTANT
>
> If you have symptoms that indicate you might have a yeast infection in your penis or genital area, treatment is easy and effective. In many cases over the counter creams and ointments will clear up the yeast infection.

After all, it is the same yeast, no matter if the host is a man or a woman. There are also some home remedies such as eating active culture yogurt which can help the body establish the proper bacteria balance. However, if home treatment does not work promptly, seek medical advice from your doctor. Your physician can determine if the symptoms are, in fact, a male yeast infection and not another more serious problem. A doctor can also prescribe strong medication to treat stubborn yeast infections in men.

Cure Male Yeast Infection Quickly with These Natural Home Remedies

Male yeast infections often respond to home remedies and natural therapies. Because this type of bacteria overabundance can not survive in less than optimal environments, all male yeast infection home remedy treatments and natural cures focus on creating an environment that will make the yeast bacteria unwelcome, removing the factors which allow the yeast to flourish.

The male yeast infection home remedies and natural treatments are the same ones used by women to treat vaginal yeast infections at home. Just because the bacteria are present as a penile infection does not mean that the treatment must be different. It simply means that the yeast has become present in the male genitals.

One effective male yeast infection home remedy is consuming yogurt with active cultures. The active cultures in yogurt provide the human body with good bacteria which allows the male body to reestablish the health balance of bacteria normally present. If yogurt is distasteful for you, the same results can be obtained by consuming dietary supplements which contain these cultures. Acidophilus is one such dietary supplement which can be purchased in capsules and other forms which have little or no taste.

Boric acid provides another natural home remedy for male yeast infection. Simply add about 2 tablespoons of boric acid to a shallow bath of water. Sit in the water for 15 minutes daily for seven days. This is a very inexpensive treatment. Do not use the boric acid bath for bathing the entire body. Use only as a sitz bath for soaking the lower body. Rinse well after soaking with clear water.

Tea tree oil can be diluted and applied to affected areas daily. The best way to use this male yeast infection natural home remedy is to prepare a shallow bath of warm water and add several drops of tea tree oil. Sit in the bath, soaking the lower body, including the genitals in the water for 15 to 20 minutes daily for several days or until symptoms are relieved.

Hydrogen peroxide can be used as a home treatment for male yeast infection. The normal 3% hydrogen peroxide which is probably already in your medicine cabinet can be used by mixing one teaspoon with one cup of water. Use a clean white face cloth wet with this solution to wash the genital area, focusing on allowing the liquid to soak the penis and glan. Use a fresh mixture each time and apply two to three times daily for up to one week or until after all symptoms have disappeared.

Potassium sorbate is a fungicide used in preserving foods which can be used as a male yeast infection home remedy. It is also used in brewing beer to stop the yeast growth at the proper time in the brewing process. You can find this product at your superstore or a specialty store which carries home brewing supplies. Mix one tablespoon of potassium sorbate with one cup of warm water. Wash genitals with a clean white cloth soaked with this mixture. Repeat two or three times daily for several days.

Male yeast infection home remedies and natural treatments are great for treating most cases. However, sometimes a yeast infection in a man can be quite stubborn.

If home remedies or natural treatments do not solve the problem, a man can use male yeast infection creams which contain non-prescription medications. If these still do not solve the problem quickly, it is imperative that advice from a qualified health care professional be sought.

Male Yeast Infection - Why It Happens and How to Avoid It

It is not uncommon for a man to experience a male yeast infection. Yeast bacteria get into the penis and result in itching, burning, pain on urination, and possibly penile discharge. Sometimes, males can have this disorder without experiencing any symptoms of any kind.

Any male, regardless of age or sexual activity can get this disorder but it is more common in sexually active men and in men who practice certain sexual behaviors. However, a young child can get a male yeast infection without having experienced any sexual contact of any kind.

Most frequently, men get yeast infections from having unprotected sex with a female partner who already has an overgrowth of vaginal yeast bacteria. This means that a yeast infection can be a sexually transmitted disease (STD), yet unlike many STDs, this is not the only means of getting the infection.

When monogamous couples practice unprotected sexual intercourse, if the female has a vaginal yeast infection, some of the bacteria can get into the opening of the penis, permitting these bacteria to multiply and resulting in an infection. While the female may obtain treatment and get better after only a few days, if the male partner is not also treated, it is quite common that the very next sexual encounter will result in the passing of the infection back to the woman. This can become a cycle until both partners are properly treated.

A male child, especially a boy baby, can easily get a yeast infection in the event that feces contact the penis. The bacteria present in feces can get into the penis and result in an infection of yeast. A boy can also get an outbreak because of being in damp clothing which provides the perfect environment for yeast bacteria to multiply into an infection.

Male Yeast Infection Cures: Which Ones Should I Use?

Male yeast infection cures can be confusing. There is far too little information available for men who may be facing this problem, leaving them wondering which cures they should use and which ones should be avoided. It seems that most available information focuses on women and vaginal yeast infections.

Men deserve accurate, helpful information on this important subject. Here, you will find the facts about male yeast infection cures that really work. Of course, the best way to cure this type of infection is to avoid getting the yeast infection in the first place, but at times, the bacteria in the body get out of balance and yeast bacteria over-multiply causing a man to experience some annoying symptoms.

If a man walks into a pharmacy or searches the over the counter pharmacy section of a store, you will find no products labels as being manufactured for treating male yeast infections! You will, however, find many products labeled for treating vaginal yeast problems, relieving symptoms of yeast infections for females, creams, ointments, vaginal suppositories, medication-filled capsules for inserting into the vagina to treat this problem. But nothing is clearly labels as being right for a man to use if he has signs and symptoms of a male yeast infection or penile yeast infection.

Itching of the genitals can be a problem for men during a yeast infection. The creams and ointments available over the counter for female itching of the vulva and labia can be used just as effectively by men. Just apply the product to the affected areas as frequently as recommended by the package. These products can be very effective for relieving the itching and burning of surface tissue associated with a male yeast infection.

Products which contain over the counter medication to treat vaginal yeast infections that use a cream to be inserted into a plunger applicator for vaginal infections are just as useful for curing male yeast infections. Apply the cream freely to the penis, and if there are signed that yeast is affecting the scrotum and other genital areas, apply the cream there as well. These products are best used at bedtime and clean underwear should be worn to prevent the cream from getting onto bed linens. Use these creams for the period of time indicated on the package, simply ignoring the instruction about inserting the product into the plunger application and into the vagina. Instead, apply with clean hands or sterile gauze pads.

Acidophilus dietary supplements or foods with active bacterial cultures like yogurt or buttermilk can be consumed and often will cure male yeast infections in mild cases. A natural cure that also works well is washing the genitals with yogurt diluted in water and leaving the yogurt on the skin overnight; again, this should be applied with clean hands or sterile gauze and clean white underwear should be worn to prevent linen stains. This cure works because the good bacteria in the yogurt fight the overgrowth of yeast bacteria.

In cases of male yeast infection where symptoms are severe or if there is no response to over the counter treatment or natural home remedies, it is important that a man talk to his health care professional about the problem.

Symptoms of a male yeast infection, in a few cases, could indicate a more serious problem such as a sexually transmitted disease (STD) such as gonorrhea or syphilis. Any yeast infection which doesn't respond quickly to treatment should be accessed by a doctor. Once the yeast infection is confirmed, a doctor can prescribe much stronger treatments than those available over the counter or at home. These may include oral medication or prescription-strength creams or ointments.

The Three Best Ways to Treat Male Yeast Infections

Male yeast infections require treatment just as do yeast infections in females. However, men will find no section of products in their local drug store that indicate they are to be used by men for this problem. This can leave a man discouraged and depressed because of annoying symptoms and no apparent treatments.

Do not despair! There are effective male yeast infection treatments available in your local stores; they just are not labels in a way that a man can easily locate them. A man has to know what he is looking for in order to locate one of the three best ways to treat male yeast infections.

The most convenient, easy to use, and effective male yeast infection treatment is found on the shelves labels as cream for vaginal yeast infections. Products which contain miconazole or clotrimazole are the best choices. Compare labels because you may find that some brands are much less expensive yet contains the same quantity of the active ingredient as more expensive brands. Look for products that are cream or ointments to be applied using a plunger applicator which is filled with the cream for each use. Do not select products that have the medication encapsulated in a gelatin capsule or are in the form of hard suppositories since these delivery methods do not lend themselves to use by a male.

The next of the three best ways to treat male yeast infections is simply a dietary choice. Because the bacteria which cause a penile yeast infection or male yeast infection that affects the genital area have over-multiplied from the numbers normally present in the hu man body, consuming yogurt, smoothies, buttermilk or other products which contain active cultures can cure the infection by restoring the natural balance. The good bacteria in active cultures work to control the number of yeast present, resulting in a cure. Some people find these foods distasteful and prefer to take a dietary supplement which contains acidophilus.

A natural home remedy that is very effective in mild cases of male yeast infection, especially when the infection symptoms involve itchy, flaky skin on the male genitals involves creating an environment in which the yeast bacteria do not thrive by changing the skin pH. Mixing boric acid with water in a shallow bath works great for most male yeast infections. Add two tablespoons of boric acid to a warm sitz bath about three inches in depth, just deep enough to soak the genital area well. This is a treatment in which more is not better. Do not add too much boric acid or it can cause dry skin, irritation and other side effects and the pH provided by the recommended mixture is sufficient to discourage the yeast bacteria overpopulation.

If none of the three best ways to treat male yeast infections work in a stubborn case, you should talk to your doctor who can prescribe medication effective in cases that require super-strength treatment to obtain a cure of the male yeast infection.

During treatment for male yeast infection, be sure you do not pass the infection to your sex partner. In fact, you may well have gotten the infection from a partner with a yeast infection. It is quite common for partners who practice unprotected sex to pass yeast bacteria back and forth, resulting in an seemingly chronic infection. Instead, both partners should treat their yeast infections and abstain from sex for a few days until both are free of all symptoms. If you wish to have sex during treatment, use protection but some men have found that use of a latex condom that is treated with noxinol-9 can be irritating during an active infection.

Three Top Causes of Male Yeast Infection

By knowing the top three causes of male yeast infection, it is much easier for a man to avoid getting an infection or passing infection back and forth with his partner. As with any infection or illness, prevention is the best possible treatment!

In order to understand the causes of yeast infections, it is important to understand the infection itself. Yeast bacteria are normally present in the human body, both in the digestive tract and sexual organs, but in limited numbers. There are other bacteria normally present in the body which are called good bacteria. These good bacteria work to restrict the less desirable bacteria to healthy levels so that they do not become too abundant. A male yeast infection, just like a female yeast infection, occurs when this balance gets out of whack.

The single most common cause of male yeast infection is unprotected sexual activity with a partner who has a yeast infection. In fact, partners can pass the yeast infection back and forth so unless both partners are treated, it can turn into a seemingly endless cycle.

Another common cause of male yeast infection is taking prescription antibiotics. Tetracycline is a common culprit but other antibiotics can have the same result. This is because antibiotics indiscriminately kill bacteria, both good and bad ones. This sets up a situation where the yeast bacteria can overwhelm the good bacteria.

Yet another cause of male yeast infection is undetected or uncontrolled diabetes.

Because yeast bacteria thrive on sugar and uncontrolled diabetes causes too much sugar to be in the body, this can result in rampant yeast growth.

These are the three most common causes of male yeast infections. There are a few other suggested causes, but many of them are not proven; for example, some people say that drinking too much beer causes yeast infection in men because of the yeast in beer. This, however, is not scientifically proven.

Twenty Most Common Signs and Symptoms of Male Yeast Infection and a Simple Test

Male yeast infection is a topic that is not discussed widely. Too frequently, information focuses on vaginal yeast infections and fails to address the fact that males can experience penile yeast infection as well as yeast infections on other parts of the male genitals.

When a man gets a yeast infection he may experience no symptoms at all. But often there are symptoms which may not cause the male to think that the cause is yeast at all. The symptoms may or may not involve the penis or genital area.

Symptoms of Male Yeast Infection Involving Penis and Genitals

- The major symptoms involving the male genitalia which may indicate a male yeast infection can be the same as symptoms which can indicate a much more serious sexually transmitted disease (STD) such as syphilis. However, the simple test provided at the end of this article can help determine if yeast is the culprit. The symptoms are:
- Glan, the head of the penis, may become red and inflamed.
- Urination may be slightly painful. This symptom usually do not cause the severe pain associated with more serious STDs but can be annoying. This symptom can also indicate a urinary tract infection.
- Jock itch may develop in the genital area.
- The male may experience sexual dysfunction not normally experienced.

Symptoms of Male Yeast Infection Not Involving Genitals

Here we will continue the list of symptoms, but focus on symptoms and signs which do not involve the genitals, often causing the man to fail to identify the source of the problem:

- Digestive problems may appear because of the lack of intestinal flora balance due to the over growth of yeast.
- Constipation may occur.
- Bad breath may appear even though good oral hygiene is practiced.
- Bloating due to yeast bacteria over-growth in the digestive tract may appear.
- Frequent intestinal gas is another indication of the yeast imbalance.
- Diarrhea may be a sign of male yeast infection.
- Loose stools may be present but no actual diarrhea.
- Irritability due to general health changes are common.
- Mood swings in a man who does not normally experience mood swings can be a sign of male yeast infection.
- Abnormal fatigue without unusual levels of activity may signal an infection.
- Lack of energy in a male who is normally energetic can be a sign of a yeast outbreak.
- Memory loss is sometimes a symptom.
- Unusually dry, flaky skin which is itchy can indicate yeast growth.
- Athlete foot outbreaks, caused by similar bacteria can be indicative of a male yeast infection.
- Sudden onset of prostate-like problems such as frequent urination urges may be present.
- An unusual craving for sweets or carbohydrates because the yeast bacteria want to be fed.

Simple Test for Male Yeast Infections

This is a very simple, easy to perform test to help a man determine if the signs and symptoms he may be experiencing are in fact caused by a yeast infection. To prepare for the test, simply place a glass of water next to the bed before retiring for the night.

Upon awakening, before getting out of bed, spit into the glass of water two times. During the next 15 minutes, watch the saliva in the water carefully. If the saliva dissipates into the water, there is most likely no yeast infection. But, if the saliva becomes cloudy, stringy, sinks to the bottom of the glass, or takes on an appearance of spider webs, there is most likely a male yeast infection present in the man's body.

The appearance of these saliva indications is very noticeable, so a man with a yeast infection will have no difficulty recognizing the signs. Do not worry that the signals may be unclear. Usually, within the first five minutes, it will be very clear whether indicators of yeast infection are present.

What Creams Should I Use to Treat Male Yeast Infection?

A male yeast infection requires treatment, but a man who walks into a pharmacy and looks for creams to treat male yeast infection will find nothing available. So, what is a man to do to treat an outbreak of yeast?

The bacteria which cause male yeast infections are the exact same bacteria present in vaginal yeast infections. In fact, quite often the man got the yeast infection from coming in contact with his sexual partner who had an active vaginal yeast infection. The same creams used by women for vaginal yeast infection can be used by men for treating male yeast infection!

On any pharmacy or superstore shelves, a man can locate products which indicate they are for use by women for yeast infections. Some of these products are in suppository form or gel capsules meant to dissolve inside the vagina. While these products contain the same medication the male needs, they are not in the right form for use on the male sex organs. Along side these products will be several choices of creams or ointments which are packaged with a plunger device for a woman to insert the cream into the vagina. These are the products a man needs for treating his penile yeast infection.

One type of product that is effective for male yeast infection is a cream which contains miconazole nitrate. Another effective male yeast infection cream is one that contains clotrimazole. These medications are found in any number of over the counter creams which a male can use to treat a yeast infection.

To effectively use the male yeast infection cream, simple ignore the instruction which indicate the cream must be inserted into the vagina. Instead, apply the cream to the penis and effective areas of the genital region. The instruction will, however, indicate how many applications must be used to treat the infection. Use the cream for male yeast infection treatment for the length of time recommended.

In the event that male yeast infection cream does not cure the problem, a man can first try the cream which contains different active ingredients. For instance, if the initial treatment was with a cream containing miconazole nitrate, then try clotrimazole cream. If, after trying both medications available over the counter for male yeast infections, there has been no improvement, it is time to seek the advice of your doctor.

What is the Best Cure for Male Yeast Infections?

Male yeast infections can be annoying, painful, and no man wants to experience yeast infections. But it is a fact of life at, at time a man may well experience just this problem. What should a man do if he knows he has contracted a yeast infection? What is the best medicine for yeast infections of the male genitalia?

Mild cases of yeast infections in men can often be cured by using natural remedies. Acidophilus and active cultures in yogurt, buttermilk and nutritional supplements can be consumed to help the natural balance of bacteria be restores. A yeast infection, whether experience by a man or woman, is really just an imbalance of bacteria naturally present in the human body. Good bacteria normally keep the number of yeast bacteria at a normal level, but when the yeast bacteria flourish and over-multiply, it is referred to as a yeast infection or yeast outbreak.

When a man is prescribed antibiotics because of some type of infection, perhaps a sinus infection or upper respiratory infection, the antibiotics attack the bacteria in the body. The drug kills the bacteria causing the medical condition, but also kills good bacteria which maintain a healthy balance of flora in the human body. By being proactive, male yeast infections prompted by taking prescription antibiotics can often be avoided by adding extra yogurt or acidophilus supplements to the diet, helping replace the good bacteria so that yeast can not multiply out of control.

When a man experiences yeast that causes the head of the penis, the glan, to redden and itch, or other genital areas to become itchy, use of readily available over the counter creams and ointments made for treating vaginal yeast infections can successfully treat the yeast outbreak. The yeast which causes vaginal infections is the same ones that can cause penile yeast infections. Simply apply the product to the affected areas for the duration recommended; simply ignore the instructions which indicate the product should only be inserted into the vagina.

Should symptoms of male yeast infection persist and fail to respond to home treatment, it is imperative that the advice of a qualified health care professional be sought. There are some much more serious sexually transmitted diseases which can have symptoms similar to those of a male yeast infection but which require much different treatment in order to cure the disease.

When experiencing any symptoms of penile yeast infection, either abstain from sexual activity or practice only protected sex. It is quite easy to transmit the yeast infection to your partner. If you have a committed relationship, sometimes it is best if both partners treat the yeast infection at the same time to prevent passing the yeast infection from the male to the partner and back again, resulting in a cycle that seems as if treatment is not effective, when in fact, re-infection is the cause of the lack of improvement.

Natural Remedies for Yeast Infections That Work Fast!

A yeast infection can be an unpleasant experience and treated promptly, whether it occurs in a male or female. Babies or children of either gender can get these infections, without any type of sexual contact as can in adults of either gender.

There are natural remedies for a yeast infection which can be very effective. One that really works is to consume yogurt or other food products with natural, active cultures. The lactobacillus acidophilus in the food provides good bacteria to prevent the overgrowth of the yeast bacteria in the vagina or penis. Regular consumption of food with active cultures can ward off chronic infection as well as improve your overall digestive health. This natural treatment works for both males and females.

A tampon soaked in a mixture created by adding one tablespoon of potassium sorbate, inserted and left in overnight can be effective. Boric acid, inserted into empty gelatin capsules obtained from a pharmacist and used as vaginal suppositories, is recommended by many natural remedy experts. Tea tree oil, applied to the top half of a tampon applicator along with some lubricant such as KY Jelly, can also be used as a natural treatment for yeast infections. These remedies are used for several days, until symptoms vanish.

A douche of one teaspoon hydrogen peroxide plus one cup of water, used daily until the symptoms disappear can often solve the infection. One to two tablespoons of white vinegar in one cup of water douched daily can create vaginal environment sufficiently acidic to cause the bacteria to return to normal levels. Lemon juice or vita min C (ascorbic acid) also provides an acidic douche mixture.

A more complex but effective douche can be made by adding several tablespoons of tea created from the following recipe to water and using every other day or daily for severe infection:

- One part of raspberry or comfrey leaf
- One part sage
- One-quarter part goldenseal.
- Steep four tablespoons of herbs in one quart of boiling water for about 20 minutes
- Strain and cool to room temperature, then add:
- Two tablespoons white vinegar
- One-fourth cup of yogurt or acidophilus powder

Be aware that any natural remedy which treats a female but not her sexual partner may allow re-infection during sex. Both partners must address the yeast infection to ensure it is not passed back and forth repeatedly if unprotected sexual intercourse occurs.

Free Downloadable Bonus Reports

As another way to express our gratitude we want to give you six - free valuable reports.

All you have to do is go to the webpage listed below and instantly download your reports.

There is no catch. This is our way of saying thanks!

Your free reports include:

- Yeast Infection Questionnaire and Score Sheet
- Skyrocket Your Fat-Loss!
- The Healing Power Of Water
- How and When to Be Your Own Doctor
- The Complete Handbook of Nature's Cures
- Lessons From The Miracle Doctors

Download your free reports by going to:

www.MaleYeastInfectionCures.com/freereports.htm